THE ULTIMATE GUIDE
CBD
— HEMP OIL —

HOW TO BUY CANNABIDIOL OIL AND CHOOSE THE RIGHT PRODUCT FOR PAIN RELIEF, ANXIETY, DEPRESSION, PARKINSON'S DISEASE, ARTHRITIS, CANCER, ADHD AND INSOMNIA

THC FREE

PAUL WHITE

CBD Hemp Oil

THE ULTIMATE GUIDE. HOW TO BUY CANNABIDIOL OIL AND CHOOSE THE RIGHT PRODUCT FOR PAIN RELIEF, ANXIETY, DEPRESSION, PARKINSON'S DISEASE, ARTHRITIS, CANCER, ADHD AND INSOMNIA

THC FREE

© **Copyright 2019 - All rights reserved.**

The content contained within this book may not be reproduced, duplicated or transmitted without direct written permission from the author or the publisher.

Under no circumstances will any blame or legal responsibility be held against the publisher, or author, for any damages, reparation, or monetary loss due to the information contained within this book. Either directly or indirectly.

Legal Notice:
This book is copyright protected. This book is only for personal use. You cannot amend, distribute, sell, use, quote or paraphrase any part, or the content within this book, without the consent of the author or publisher.

Disclaimer Notice:
Please note the information contained within this document is for educational and entertainment purposes only. All effort has been executed to present accurate, up to date, and reliable, complete information. No warranties of any kind are declared or implied. Readers acknowledge that the author is not engaging in the rendering of legal, financial, medical or professional advice. The content within this book has been derived from various sources. Please consult a licensed professional before attempting any techniques outlined in this book.

By reading this document, the reader agrees that under no circumstances is the author responsible for any losses, direct or indirect, which are incurred as a result of the use of information contained within this document, including, but not limited to, — errors, omissions, or inaccuracies.

Table of Content

Introduction 1

Chapter 1: What CBD Oil is and How it Works 4

    History of CBD Oil 5

    What Is CBD Oil? 7

    The Chemistry And Biology of CBD: How it Works 8

    Difference Between CBD Oil and Hemp Oil 11

        What is Hemp Oil? 12

        Uses of Hemp Oil 13

    Benefits of CBD Oil 14

        Pain Relief 15

        Quit Smoking 16

        Treat Epilepsy 17

        Reduce Anxiety 17

        Cancer Treatment 18

        Treat Type 1 Diabetes 19

        Treat Alzheimer's Disease 19

        Loss of Appetite and Nausea 20

        Enhancing Cardiovascular Health 21

        Sleep and Insomnia 22

        Promote Healthy Weight 22

        CBD For Skin Care and Acne 23

        CBD for Attention Deficit Disorder (ADHD) 23

        CBD For Depression 24

    CBD Oil Vs. Standard Pain Medication 25

Does CBD Oil Get You High? 27

Is It Safe? Is Medical Supervision Necessary? 29

Is It Legal? 30

Where is CBD Illegal? 31

Will CBD Oil Appear on A Drug Test? 32

    Product With THC 33

    Mislabeling of Products 33

    Cross Contamination of THC 34

    Passive Exposure to THC 34

    Tricks to Pass a CBD Drug Test 34

Chapter 2: Methods of Usage and What to Use it For 36

    Tincture Consumption 36

    Ingestion 37

    Topical Applications 37

    Smoking/Inhaling 38

CBD Dosage: How Much Should You Take? 38

Choosing An Ideal CBD Dosage 40

    Use Your Body Weight to Decide 40

    Know The Concentration of CBD Oil 41

    Desired Effects 41

    Tolerance 42

    Talk to Your Physician 42

How Much is Too Much? 42

CBD Side Effects 43

Disorders and Diseases 44

    Multiple Sclerosis 44

    Spinal Cord Injury 45

Arthritis 45

Epilepsy 45

High Blood Pressure 46

Diabetes 47

Chapter 3: How to Buy CBD Oil: Finding the Right Product 48

Packaging 48

Price of CBD 49

Top CBD Brands 49

Compare Strength 50

Source of CBD Product 51

Flavor 51

Other Ingredients 51

Health Claims 52

Quality Testing 52

Go Through Reviews 52

CBD Oil Recipes 53

CBD Chamomile Tea Latte 53

CBD Bliss Balls 54

Final Thoughts 56

Bibliography 63

Introduction

There are certain diseases that have become a normal thing for most people in today's world. When you talk about diseases such as insomnia, depression, anxiety, diabetes, cancer, arthritis, and chronic pains, these are common diseases. Previously, people had all sorts of methods of dealing with such diseases. To some extent, medical experts have in the past recommended engaging in regular exercise to help in preventing and reducing the effects of such ailments. Today, all this has changed with the recent legalization of marijuana.

Chances are, you're probably wondering how cannabis products could help you in living a healthier and happier life. Undeniably, few people understand how marijuana can be used as medicine instead of an abused drug. With the recent legalization of marijuana, CBD surged in popularity and dominated the market as one of the best remedies for the mentioned diseases. To clearly understand its health benefits, you have to comprehend what the product is.

So, what exactly is CBD? CBD is an acronym for cannabidiol[1]. Cannabidiol is found in the cannabis plant. It is one of the many compounds that can be extracted from the plant. CBD

---

[1] "CBD oil: Uses, health benefits, and risks - Medical News Today." 27 Jul. 2018, https://www.medicalnewstoday.com/articles/317221.php. Accessed 19 Apr. 2019.

oils are those which are extracted from CBD. It is worth noting that the concentration of CBD in these oils varies. Equally, the uses are also distinct.

One of the main questions that must be lingering in your mind is; is CBD marijuana? Well, initially, researchers only knew that the best compound in cannabis was delta-9 tetrahydrocannabinol (THC)[2]. It is considered as a dominant ingredient in marijuana. Marijuana has two compounds, CBD and THC. The compounds have very different effects on the body. When an individual claims that they are "high," this is the effect of THC. The effect of CBD on the body is different. CBD does not have any psychoactive effects on the body. This implies that one cannot claim that they are feeling high after using CBD. Regardless, CBD has effects on the body which are considered to be important. Having said this, CBD is not marijuana, but it is a compound found in the plant. It has positive health effects on the body and it doesn't pose any psychoactive effects.

Unfortunately, few people understand what CBD is. This creates a challenge to most individuals that would want to use the product to address diseases such as arthritis, sleep disorders, and more. If you have been meaning to use CBD and you haven't found the right information to help you search

---

[2] "CBD oil: Uses, health benefits, and risks - Medical News Today."

for the right product, this is the right book for you. With the help of this guide, you will learn how to choose the best CBD oil on the market. Additionally, this book will provide tips on some of the healthiest ways of using the product. Besides this, you will garner deeper insight into the positive health effects of using CBD oil. Just like any other prescription, this material will also point out to you its side effects.

Undeniably, when medicine is used in the properly prescribed way, there is a high possibility of recovering from a disease that you have been suffering from. This means that for CBD to work, you have to follow the recommended dosages. Don't just take the product because it helps you relieve pain or it soothes you to sleep. You have to stick to the recommended dosages for effective results.

Bearing in mind that there are numerous associated health benefits of using cannabidiol, the best move to take is to learn how to use the product. This product can be ingested in many ways including through inhaling, capsules, sprays, edibles, dabbing, strips, etc. However, medical experts argue that the best way of getting good results from CBD is by using CBD oil. It is for this reason that this book will focus on CBD oil and how it can help your body.

Chapter 1: What CBD Oil is and How it Works

Many might think that CBD is a product that was recently introduced after marijuana was legalized in several states in the U.S. But this isn't the case. CBD dates back to about 4000 years ago[3]. People have been cultivating cannabis for a very long time. The only issue is that the product had not been legalized until recently. More on the history of cannabidiol will be looked at in this section. This chapter will also explain further what CBD oil is and how it functions.

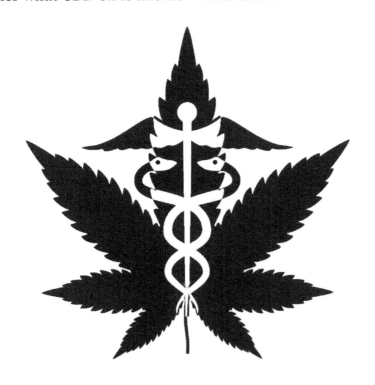

---

[3] "The Brief History of CBD - PureRatiosHoldings - Pure Ratios CBD." https://www.pureratioscbd.com/blogs/news/the-brief-history-of-cbd. Accessed 19 Apr. 2019.

History of CBD Oil

Over the past few years, CBD oil has become well known for being an ideal remedy for numerous diseases. Part of the main reason for this is due to its minimal side effects. Also, the product is the number one choice for most users because it is obtained naturally. With this information, you might jump to the conclusion that CBD was recently introduced. CBD has been here for ages. The only thing that is happening differently today is that people are beginning to understand how CBD works with the body.

The earliest records of cannabis use can be dated back to 6000 B.C. This was in ancient China during the onset of human civilization[4]. However, reliable evidence of cannabis use began to show up around 2700 B.C. Back in 2737 B.C., a Chinese emperor named Shen-Nung was recorded to have used cannabis to aid in treating pain[5]. With time, people moved towards civilization and writings documenting the importance of cannabis appeared across Asia. At first, the writings of Hua Tuo documented the use of cannabis as an anesthetic and blood thinner. This was recorded during the second century B.C.

Later, in A.D. 77, the Romans adopted the idea of using hemp widely. Some early writings by one of the Roman scholars

---

[4] "2019 Ultimate Guide to CBD Oil: What is It? How Does ... - Joy Organics." https://joyorganics.com/ultimate-guide-to-cbd-oil/. Accessed 24 Apr. 2019.
[5] "2019 Ultimate Guide to CBD Oil: What is It? How Does ... - Joy Organics."

called Pliny the Elder revealed that cannabis aided in pain relief.

Things were no different in the West. By the 16th century, cannabis had become well-known and was cultivated throughout Europe. At the time, hemp was regarded as highly important. In fact, in 1533, Henry VIII ordered all farmers to embrace the idea of growing hemp.

In modern times, people began the manufacture of modern medicines including opioids. The introduction of these medicines in the 20th century led to the decline in the use of cannabis as a pain reliever. Nevertheless, there were medications which still used cannabis as an ingredient, such as sleep aids, cough syrups, and other pharmaceuticals.

By the late 1930s, cultivation of cannabis faced a huge challenge when it was considered illegal[6]. The worst occurred in 1970 after its cultivation was banned by the passing of the Controlled Substance Act. This law listed hemp and cannabis as substances that had no proven medical benefits. It also pointed out that the plants posed a high risk of dependence.

In spite of the legal restrictions, cannabis was still used by many for healing purposes. About a century later, the State of California authorized the use of cannabis for medicinal purposes only. At the time, it listed a number of serious

---

[6] "2019 Ultimate Guide to CBD Oil: What is It? How Does ... - Joy Organics." https://joyorganics.com/ultimate-guide-to-cbd-oil/. Accessed 24 Apr. 2019.

medical conditions which cannabis could be used for.

Since then, numerous studies have looked into the health benefits of cannabinoids and, more specifically, CBD benefits. The vast media coverage of CBD is what has contributed to its huge acceptance in the United States. The good news that CBD has various health benefits is gradually reaching more and more people.

Today, CBD oil can conveniently be accessed by everyone. Whether you choose to purchase CBD over the internet or in conventional stores, you can easily get it. The best part is that there is continued research that is unveiling how CBD can be beneficial to the body.

What Is CBD Oil?

An individual that knows little about CBD oil would easily conclude that CBD oil is marijuana. Scientifically, this is not true. Arguing that CBD is marijuana would only mean that it has psychoactive properties; something that is far from the truth. CBD (cannabidiol) is one of the compounds in the Cannabis plant[7]. The product can be consumed in several ways including tinctures, vaping, edibles, and capsules. Another component found in Cannabis is called tetrahydrocannabinol (THC). This is the compound responsible for the "high" feeling

---

[7] "CBD101: The CBD Beginner's Guide – CBD Origin – Medium." 30 Jul. 2018, https://medium.com/cbd-origin/cbd101-the-cbd-beginners-guide-986274bbdf1b. Accessed 19 Apr. 2019.

that one gains when smoking marijuana.

Just to clear the air; a patient using CBD would not get stoned. This is because CBD lacks the psychoactive properties that THC has. Therefore, CBD and THC have different effects on the body. Part of the main reason why many people are switching to CBD is because of the harsh side effects of using over the counter drugs. Consequently, drugs that are in sync with nature are more preferred. A recommended use of CBD would help a lot in relieving anxiety, chronic pain, depression, inflammation, and several other conditions.

Through extensive research, medics argue that CBD can be used to treat numerous diseases including:

- Autoimmune diseases
- Neurological diseases
- Neuropsychiatric diseases
- Gut disorders
- Skin diseases

More on this will be discussed later in this material.

The Chemistry And Biology of CBD: How it Works

After pointing out that CBD will not get you stoned, you might be asking yourself how this is possible. A look into the chemical and biological properties of the component will help in understanding this. The molecular structure of CBD and THC reveals the fact that the two compounds are different from each other. This is the main reason why they have varying properties and effects on the body.

One thing you ought to know is that THC and CBD have a similar chemical makeup. Both compounds have:

- 21 carbon atoms

- 30 hydrogen atoms

- 2 oxygen atoms

Now, you must be wondering how these two are different and yet have similar chemical properties. Well, the difference lies in the arrangement of their atoms. This is depicted in the image below.

Cannabidiol   Tetrahydrocannabinol

Source: "CBD vs THC: The Difference Explained – CBD Origin – Medium."[8]

If you have a good memory from your chemistry class, you should remember the meaning of an atom. In comparison to the human hair, an atom is a million times smaller. Consequently, there is a microscopic disparity between CBD and THC. This microscopic difference is what causes the products to differ.

Cannabidiol and tetrahydrocannabinol are not the only cannabinoid compounds constituted in the cannabis plant. There are about 85 of them. However, the most popular are CBD and THC[9]. What is a cannabinoid? This refers to a compound which reacts with the Endocannabinoid System (ECS) of the body. Simply said, it is a network of receptors interacting with cannabinoids to ensure that vital functions of the body are maintained. The first cannabinoid receptor was discovered by scientists in 1988. Later, a second receptor was discovered in 1993[10]. These receptors are identified as CB1 and CB2.

With the varying molecular structures of CBD and THC, this affects their interaction with the mentioned receptors. It is for

---

[8] "CBD vs THC: The Difference Explained – CBD Origin – Medium." 29 Sep. 2018, https://medium.com/cbd-origin/cbd-vs-thc-the-difference-explained-b3cfc1da52f0. Accessed 19 Apr. 2019.
[9] "CBD vs THC: The Difference Explained – CBD Origin – Medium.".
[10] "CBD vs THC: The Difference Explained – CBD Origin – Medium."

this reason that they have varying effects on the body. The varying effects that CBD and THC have on the body make the products also vary with regards to their legality. Most nations consider THC as an illegal substance simply because of its mind-altering attributes. The legal aspects of CBD will be looked at in detail later on.

To clearly understand how CBD works, it is important to look into the endocannabinoid system. This is a system that is essential in regulating a wide range of physiological processes including our energy levels, moods, blood pressure, stress, anger, intestinal fortitude, pain experiences, glucose metabolism, and more. By working on the endocannabinoid system, CBD helps in slowing down or stopping disease from progressing.

Difference Between CBD Oil and Hemp Oil

When planning to use CBD, you could either go for pharmaceutical CBD or CBD obtained from other internet storefronts, coffee shops, community markets, gas stations, chiropractic offices, health clubs, etc. In line with this, when out in search of natural oils, you will certainly come across CBD oil as well as hemp oil. It is important to get it clear that hemp oil and CBD oil are terms that are at times used interchangeably. Regardless, these products differ. Let's take a closer look at the distinction between the two products.

What is Hemp Oil?

Hemp oil and CBD oil differ in the sense that they come from different sources. The former is obtained from the hemp plant. The hemp plant is part of the cannabis sativa family. Often, the plant is used for industrial purposes[11]. A striking attribute of the hemp plant is that it has low levels of cannabinoids. The popular cannabinoids, CBD and THC, are also present in the hemp plant. To obtain hemp oil, the content is extracted from the seeds. When the hemp seeds are pressed, oil is produced. This process of oil extraction is similar to how coconut oil is extracted.

Interestingly, hemp seeds lack THC. This implies that the extracted content also lacks the component. Nevertheless, small quantities of THC can still be traced because the plant matter adheres to the seeds while being processed. Hemp oil extracted from the hemp plant could either contain CBD or THC. The issue is that the product might still be labeled as hemp oil just because it is obtained from the hemp plant. As such, it is crucial that you confirm that you are getting the right product from the store. Notably, if you are out looking for hemp oil containing CBD only, ensure that you confirm it's

---

[11] "Hemp Oil vs CBD Oil | What is the Difference? - Namaste.com." 15 May. 2018, https://www.namaste.com/blogs/news/hemp-oil-vs-cbd-oil-what-is-the-difference. Accessed 19 Apr. 2019.

THC-free.

While shopping for CBD oil, one should bear in mind that CBD oil could also be obtained from cannabis plants. These plants have high levels of THC. Consequently, this information is important and should be clearly labeled in the product that you purchase.

Uses of Hemp Oil

There are several ways in which hemp oil can be used. Its varying uses is part of the main reason why hemp oil has become famous in the past few years. First, the oil can be used as a food supplement. This is for the reasons that it is rich in vitamins E, B, B1, and B2[12]. It also has other nutrients including potassium, fatty acids, and magnesium. In most cases, the oil is used in soaps, lotions, shampoos, and other cosmetic products.

Hemp oil has numerous benefits, considering the fact that it has several nutrients. Hemp oil has both omega-3 and omega-6. By using this oil, one benefits from lowering their signs of aging. Equally, hemp oil helps in keeping the heart healthy. When purchasing hemp oil from the store, one should be careful about its contents. There are some oils that have some

---

[12] "Hemp Oil vs CBD Oil | What is the Difference? - Namaste.com." 15 May. 2018, https://www.namaste.com/blogs/news/hemp-oil-vs-cbd-oil-what-is-the-difference. Accessed 20 Apr. 2019.

CBD contents, and others that have none at all. It is for this reason that you are strongly advised to read the labels before making a purchase.

CBD oil and hemp oil differ not just because they have a varying extraction process. The main difference that lies between the two is evident from their intended use. CBD oil is considered to be more beneficial as compared to hemp oil. The good news about the two products is that one would not go through psychoactive effects associated with marijuana. One of the main reasons why people would choose to go for CBD oil is to help them deal with stress or pains. On the other hand, hemp oil is used on a regular basis as a supplement to gain essential nutrients from it. Therefore, hemp oil is not used to free one from stress or pain. So, it should be clear that hemp oil and CBD oil are different more so concerning their effects on the body. Don't be confused between the two. Before going for either of the two products, it is advisable to consult with your doctor. They will offer you the right guidance depending on your goals and body needs.

Benefits of CBD Oil

After understanding what CBD oil is, you need to learn more about its benefits. Equipping yourself with information aids in making sure that you purchase the oil for the right reasons.

The benefits of CBD oil will be looked at here. However, it should be known that one should seek expert consultation before trying out any cannabinoid extract.

Pain Relief

There is nothing worse than going through pain in the body. The worst thing about this is that knowing the exact source of pain could be even more challenging. As a result, getting the best treatment options is difficult. Often, this leaves an individual suffering in silence. At times, people are forced to avoid activities that they once used to enjoy.

If you have been going through significant pain, you should bear in mind that you are never alone. Yes, you might be suffering in silence, but you should be aware that there are millions out there who are sailing in the same boat. Research shows that about 11% of the general population is affected by chronic pains[13]. This pain affects their day to day lives. Pain could be the resultant effect of inflammation. Inflammation could also be the main reason why such pain worsens.

Research has shown that CBD can help in reducing such pain and providing relief. It can also help in preventing further inflammation. The use of CBD comes highly recommended

---

[13] "20 CBD Oil Benefits - Ultimate Guide on How to ... - CBD Central." 12 Apr. 2019, https://www.cbdcentral.com/cbd-ultimate-benefits-guide/. Accessed 21 Apr. 2019.

because it lacks the side effects that over the counter drugs have. Some of the side effects that these drugs pose include addiction, cardiovascular damage, liver damage, withdrawal, and more[14]. CBD does not have these side effects. How does CBD work on reducing or preventing inflammation from occurring? Well, it targets a3 glycine receptors found in the brain and the spinal cord. CBD controls how these receptors react to pain. Through its interaction with these receptors, pain sensation is considerably reduced.

Quit Smoking

Besides helping you deal with pain, CBD is also known to help people quit smoking. Smoking is a deadly health habit. It kills one slowly but surely. When one is addicted to smoking, it becomes a challenge to quit. In fact, 70% of the U.S. population has tried to quit, by they have ended up failing[15]. If you are a smoker, chances are that you have tried all the medications out there, but nothing seems to work. You should understand that there is a natural remedy to turn to; CBD oil.

It is not entirely clear yet how CBD oil helps one quit smoking, but studies have shown that addition to nicotine is closely related to the endocannabinoid system. This is a system that CBD interacts with and therefore, it could help in regulating

---

[14] "20 CBD Oil Benefits - Ultimate Guide on How to ... - CBD Central."
[15] "20 CBD Oil Benefits - Ultimate Guide on How to ... - CBD Central.".

it.

Treat Epilepsy

There are promising signs that CBD could help in treating epilepsy. There is a CBD-based drug that is approved by the FDA, Epidiolex, it is used in treating complex symptoms of epilepsy. Medical experts have researched this and have found that there is a considerable reduction in the number of seizures from patients using CBD oil. Therefore, if you know an individual that has been struggling with the disease for a long time, you could recommend CBD oil.

Reduce Anxiety

Anxiety can come in many forms. It could be that you are having phobias, panic disorder, social anxiety disorder, obsessive-compulsive disorder, or generalized anxiety disorder. All of these are forms of anxiety. Diagnosing anxiety is often a challenge, as it is accompanied by other ailments. Going through anxiety can be weakening. It affects how one handles certain activities. In fact, it could make simple tasks appear impossible.

There are conventional remedies that treat anxiety. The main challenge is that these remedies have side effects. Some of the remedies could end up leaving one depressed and addicted. In other cases, one could end up losing or gaining too much weight. These side effects should make you consider turning to CBD oil. It is a natural remedy that lacks these effects.

Cancer Treatment

We all know of someone that has been affected by cancer. This is a deadly disease that is slowly robbing us of the people we love. We are all living in the unknown. Maybe it could be you that will be suffering next (though let's hope not). With the poor lifestyles that we have adopted, we can never be too sure about our health status. Consequently, we are always advised to learn more about how to live healthy lives.

With regards to cancer, there is a dire need to find its cure as soon as possible. The treatments that are already available are not only costly, but they are inaccessible to most individuals. There are countries where people have to travel abroad to seek cancer treatment. Therefore, natural treatment would be the best solution to save lives. Before you consider CBD as another overrated remedy, let's look at some facts here.

Medical experts have recently found out that CBD could aid in enabling antiproliferative, pro-apoptotic effects which:

- Shrink tumors
- Prevent cancer cells from migrating
- Decrease the likelihood of cancer cells attaching

themselves to other structures

- Decrease the likelihood of cancer cells growing

With the above-mentioned benefits of CBD oil, it means that the oil bears the potential of becoming the best natural cancer remedy.

Treat Type 1 Diabetes

When the body fails to control blood sugar, this is what leads to type 1 diabetes. Type 1 diabetes is an autoimmune disorder. It occurs when the immune system destroys cells within the pancreas. This leaves the body incapable of producing insulin that would have helped in controlling blood sugar. When type 1 diabetes is not controlled, it could pose serious health effects such as skin infections, cardiovascular diseases, and even brain damage. Therefore, this is a disease that should not be taken lightly.

CBD could help in treating this disease. CBD oil is known for regulating body functions. By regulating how the immune system functions, it could treat type 1 diabetes.

Treat Alzheimer's Disease

Alzheimer's disease is associated with negative health effects such as memory loss, feeling lost, and the inability to take care of one's self. The disease is quite common in the United States.

The lack of a known cure could lead to an increase in its prevalence over the years. Besides patients suffering from the disease, families also suffer as they watch their loved one losing their memories and failing to remember them. It is a bitter experience that no one should go through. While there is hope that there would be a cure for the disease sooner than we expected, CBD is a natural remedy that is actually promising.

The disease strikes by affecting the brain and other neuroreceptors. Available treatments only help in reducing the effects of the disease. However, they do not stop the disorder from progressing. Recent studies have revealed that fact that CBD oil could help in reducing such progression and in other cases, get rid of cognitive impairment.

Loss of Appetite and Nausea

The body cannot function optimally without essential nutrients. When we eat food, we provide the body with the nutrients that it needs to function properly to repair and heal the body from diseases. This means that a lack of these nutrients could cause the body to suffer, as diseases could easily progress.

Cannabis users claim that the plant helps them increase their appetite. Does CBD work in the same way? Yes, it does! It treats appetite challenges existing both in children and adults.

Certainly, there are other remedies to help you deal with the loss of appetite and nausea. However, you should not forget the fact that these remedies have negative side effects. As a result, CBD comes highly recommended.

Enhancing Cardiovascular Health

The risk of suffering from heart disease is quite alarming. The awareness that has been raised about heart diseases has influenced the lifestyles of many people. Individuals have opted to live active lives with the hopes of warding off heart-related ailments. One of the main reason why CBD could help in boosting cardiovascular health is because of its anti-oxidative and anti-inflammatory properties[16].

The product has also shown the possibility of reducing cardiac arrhythmias and reducing the risk of having another heart attack after suffering from the first. Equally, the mere fact that it regulates hypertension also implies that it aids in keeping the heart healthy. CBD aids in treating particular conditions that pose a huge risk of leading to heart diseases, for example anxiety, diabetes, stress, etc.. These ailments could ultimately lead to the development of cardiovascular diseases. Therefore, CBD works all-round to make sure that one's heart is healthy.

---

[16] "20 CBD Oil Benefits - Ultimate Guide on How to … - CBD Central." 12 Apr. 2019, https://www.cbdcentral.com/cbd-ultimate-benefits-guide/. Accessed 21 Apr. 2019.

Sleep and Insomnia

Aside from the many benefits that have been pointed out, CBD helps in dealing with sleep disorders. If you have been suffering from sleepless nights, this is the natural remedy for you. Your lack of sleep could be the resultant effect of chronic pain. CBD could also help in combating both your chronic pain and reduced sleep. Most importantly, it will help you in dealing with insomnia.

Lack of sleep is not just a simple matter that should be overlooked. It affects your normal body functions. It could lead to many life-threatening mistakes e.g. while at work or when driving. In the medical field, lack of sleep could affect the performance of a doctor and therefore could lead to a death. Consequently, treating sleep disorders and insomnia should never be neglected. Find a local store near you and buy CBD oil. Save yourself from making huge mistakes that might cost your life or the lives of others.

Promote Healthy Weight

CBD oil is also known to aid in maintaining a healthy body weight. This is possible because it works by ensuring that healthy blood sugar is maintained by the body. Also, it stimulates proteins and genes which help the body to easily break down fat and enhance mitochondria, which burn calories. Through these attributes of CBD, an individual consuming the product will find it easy to manage their weight.

CBD For Skin Care and Acne

If you have been suffering from acne or other skin conditions, then CBD should be the product that you purchase. Acne is a chronic skin condition that destroys the beautiful look of your face. It leaves one with pimples that seem not to disappear. Truly, living with a chronic skin condition is frustrating since it lowers one's self-esteem. In extreme cases, it could lead to depression. Most people opt for laser treatments and prescription products to treat such conditions. However, these treatments have their own negative effects. With CBD, you can maintain healthy skin and treat acne without facing these negative effects. Consequently, the oil comes highly recommended.

CBD for Attention Deficit Disorder (ADHD)

Another reason why CBD oil is important is because it helps in treating attention deficit disorder (ADHD). This is a disorder that begins when one is still a toddler. School-aged children could portray symptoms such as low frustration tolerance, hot temper, poor planning, impulsiveness, restlessness, and disorganization, etc. These symptoms could likely indicate that a child is suffering from ADHD. In such cases, CBD oil could be used to reduce the effects of such conditions.

The condition could easily progress to adulthood if not managed properly. An adult suffering from ADHD will find a challenge attending to day to day activities. For instance, it could affect your performance at work and your personal relationships. Accordingly, this is a condition that needs to be controlled and treated. Using CBD oil will help a lot. As earlier mentioned, CBD interacts with neurotransmitters in the brain. Therefore, it helps reduce anxiety while increasing the brain's capacity to focus. In the long run, it aids in reducing ADHD symptoms.

CBD For Depression

Most people go through depression without actually knowing that they are depressed. Depression causes a major issue when it continues for an extended period of time. Depression can be associated with several negative feelings including feeling guilty, irritable, frustrated, disappointed, sad, and miserable. The negative health effects of depression include weight gain, insomnia, appetite changes, dry mouth, and sexual effects. Regular use of CBD oil will help in dealing with these effects.

CBD Oil Vs. Standard Pain Medication

With the wide array of information available over the internet, it is easy to get lost trying to discover what is good for your body. When treating pain, one has the option of using standard pain medications or simply using CBD oil. Knowing what is best for you is important, as it ensures you make the right decision. Painkillers are often recommended when one is going through pain. It could be a mild or serious pain. This will have an impact on the type of prescription drugs that would be recommended to you.

Common over the counter drugs that you might have taken before include aspirin, naproxen, and ibuprofen. In most cases, these drugs are prescribed when people have fevers or mild pains. These drugs relieve pain, however, there are negative effects that could be experienced if taken for an extended period of time. For instance, if you take aspirin for a long period, it could cause your stomach to bleed. Problems could thereafter ensue, including stomach ulcers. Equally, you might suffer from kidney damage.

If you are going through serious pain, then doctors might recommend powerful painkillers. These pain killers are termed as opioids. Such drugs are often prescribed to those that recovering from surgery or individuals living with chronic diseases such as cancer. Unfortunately, the effectiveness of opioids comes with a heavy price tag. They have serious side effects such as nausea, dizziness, depression, drowsiness, and even addiction. Their addiction effect has led to numerous deaths.

Opioids are associated with many side effects simply because they interact with several opioid receptors found in the brain. The side effects could be experienced in a way that the body fails to react quickly in a particular situation. Also, effective movements could be hindered. Having said this, driving while experiencing such side effects is dangerous.

The long-term side effects of opioids are quite devastating. These effects depend on how the drugs are consumed. An individual that injects the drugs straight to the bloodstream could face the risk of a heart attack. A major long-term effect is addiction. This occurs when a patient feels as though they need a constant supply of the painkiller to survive. Such addiction often has a negative effect on relationships.

Now, after understanding how CBD oil functions and its benefits to the body, you can make a conclusion of whether you should go for prescription drugs or choose CBD. However, there are many things that you ought to mull over before making your decision. The most important step you need to take is to consult with your doctor before making any move. Regardless, bearing in mind that CBD oil lacks serious negative effects such as addiction, it is a preferable painkiller.

In light of the question as to whether to use CBD oil over painkillers, it would be naive to claim that painkillers are not effective. These are drugs that have been tested and that have proven to help people live happier lives. Nevertheless, one should be aware of the negative effects that they might experience when using these painkillers. With this knowledge, a patient would be better informed to make the right decisions concerning the best pain remedies that they should rely on.

If you have never used CBD before, you should start by taking small doses. Determine whether the product works for you more so in relation to managing your pains. The associated benefits of CBD oil make the product worth trying.

Does CBD Oil Get You High?

After understanding that CBD oil is extracted from the cannabis plant, you probably want to know whether the oil gets you high. Indeed, it is good to know the side effects of any drug or prescription before using it. Therefore, it is vital to know whether CBD could make you high considering the fact that it is extracted from marijuana.

So, does CBD get you high? Well, no it doesn't. As earlier discussed, Cannabidiol is different from tetrahydrocannabinol. It has no psychoactive effects like tetrahydrocannabinol does. Therefore, when using it, it will not get you stoned, as some would want to say. To understand this clearly, you should remember the fact that cannabis is a complex plant which has several other cannabinoids. Tetrahydrocannabinol is one of the cannabinoids. It is distinct from CBD due to the psychoactive effects that it has on an individual.

Now, you must be wondering: if CBD doesn't make me feel high, how will I feel? This is a valid question, as you would want to know exactly what will happen when you consume CBD. Without using any scientific terms here, CBD will make you feel relaxed from the relief it will bring to your body. Simply said, the effects of CBD are mild. It only works to deal with a condition that you might be suffering from without impairing you in any way. To be clear on this question, you will not feel weird after ingesting CBD. The only good thing that you will experience is that you will notice your pains have melted away.

Some of the feelings that you might experience can be categorized as:

- Relieved
- Relaxed
- Comfortable
- Better

- Normal

- Calm

These feelings are difficult to quantify. However, that is just how CBD works. CBD functions to optimize your body functions, leaving you with a healthy state of mind. Are you still confused about whether CBD could make you feel high? Well, you shouldn't. One thing that you should bear in mind is that CBD doesn't have psychoactive effects like other cannabinoids.

Is It Safe? Is Medical Supervision Necessary?

Another question that might ring in your mind is whether CBD oil is safe. With the wide array of information that you can access over the internet, you could easily get lost without discovering whether CBD is safe or not. From the benefits that have been discussed herein, it is clear that the product is effective. Also, you are now aware of the fact that it is non-intoxicating. Therefore, it is safe to argue that CBD is safe to use. The only issue that exists with CBD is the fact that research is still underway to determine whether the product is pure enough to treat certain medical conditions including schizophrenia, anxiety, and diabetes. Concerns have been raised regarding impurities that have been found in some products being sold in the market[17]. Some of the products purchased over the internet have THC in them.

Since there are some products which have THC in them, it is advisable for an individual to talk to their doctors before using THC. Also, the fact that some of CBD uses remain largely unproven implies that consulting with your doctor is essential.

The legal nature of marijuana in different states also makes it challenging to know whether CBD oil is legal in certain states. Some states have legalized it, whereas others are still in the process of finding out whether the product is effective or not. Therefore, the murky legality aspect of CBD calls for supervision. You need to be sure that you are buying the right product in the market.

Is It Legal?

As discussed, CBD oil is beneficial. However, you should also take the time to find out whether it is legal in your state or not. There are different answers that you would get depending on where you seek information. Due to the numerous benefits of CBD, it is important to know more about its legality. The legal aspects of CBD are confusing because the product is obtained

---

[17] "CBD Oil: All the Rage, But Is It Really Safe and Effective? – WebMD." https://www.webmd.com/pain-management/news/20180507/cbd-oil-all-the-rage-but-is-it-safe-effective. Accessed 23 Apr. 2019.

from cannabis plants. It also raises concerns about the safety of the oil.

To be clear on whether CBD is legal or not, you should know that the legality would depend on where the CBD is extracted from. CBD obtained from the hemp plant is legal. It is legal in all the 50 states in the U.S. On the other hand, CBD from marijuana is not completely legal. The government categorizes hemp as a cannabis family plant containing THC in low quantities i.e. less than 0.3%. Marijuana, on the other hand, is categorized as any plant having THC quantities above 0.3%. As you can see, the main point is whether the drug is intoxicating or not. If there is more THC present in CBD oil, then it would mean that it would have a psychoactive effect. Therefore, it would be illegal.

Where is CBD Illegal?

You might also want to know the areas where CBD is illegal. CBD that has zero THC traces is not illegal in all 50 states. This was made possible after the 2018 Farm Bill was passed[18]. Some states are considered as friendly with regards to the legality of CBD. However, there are those states that still show concern about the use of the product. It is therefore important

---

[18] "Is CBD Oil Legal in all 50 states? - Hempure." https://www.hempurecbd.com/is-cbd-oil-legal-in-all-50-states/. Accessed 23 Apr. 2019.

to know whether your state fully allows the sale and use of CBD. The friendliest states include Alaska, Indiana, Kentucky, New York, Oregon, South Carolina, Utah, Tennessee, Vermont, and a few others. States with concern include Nevada, West Virginia, California, Arizona, Nebraska, Ohio, Wyoming, and Connecticut.

So, is CBD legal? Yes, it is legal to sell and consume CBD that is extracted from the hemp plant. Before taking any product that you are not sure of, it is imperative that you confirm that the product is obtained from the hemp plant. Keep it in mind that CBD obtained from marijuana is illegal federally. Again, remember to check your state's regulations before using any CBD your purchased.

Will CBD Oil Appear on A Drug Test?

The straight answer to this question is that it is unlikely. When you are being screened for employment, the obvious content that they are looking for is cannabis. This means that the test would be looking to find out whether there are any traces of THC in your blood. They will not be looking for CBD. If you take the right CBD which lacks traces of THC, then CBD will not appear on a drug test. Yes, CBD is an extract obtained from the cannabis plant. However, it will not appear in the drug test. Why? Simply stated, its chemical structure is different from THC, as has been discussed. Consequently, any test will not detect CBD, but it will detect the presence of THC.

An issue arises when you purchase the wrong product from the store thinking that it is THC-free. It therefore makes it imperative to confirm that you are buying CBD oil that is THC-free. This is the only way that you will pass a drug test. If you are using CBD for your health, there are several reasons why you could fail a CBD drug test.

Product With THC

One of the main reasons why people fail the CBD test is because they ingest CBD oil with traces of THC. Confusion happens when shopping for the right CBD product. It mostly occurs when consumers settle for low-quality products. Such products might not be accurately labelled to prevent a user from consuming CBD with some THC traces. Similarly, there are dishonest manufacturers that could claim their products lack THC and yet they have some quantities. This could also affect the possibilities of passing a CBD test.

Mislabeling of Products

Mislabelling of products is simply misleading. The oil that is extracted from hemp plant should not have traces of THC above 0.3%. However, most sellers will label their products to be THC-free and yet they have been extracted from the marijuana plant. This means that they will have THC above 0.3% in them. A user could therefore fail their test if they fail to settle for quality products that have been accurately labeled.

Cross Contamination of THC

If there are small amounts of THC within the material where CBD is extracted from, it means that the CBD oil produced will also have THC. Accordingly, the chances of failing a CBD drug test are high in such situations.

Passive Exposure to THC

It is also likely that you could fail a CBD drug test if you expose yourself to marijuana smokers for a prolonged period. Some might argue the THC amounts that one is exposed to are not enough to fail a test, but there are slight chances that it could affect your CBD drug test. Therefore, you should be wary of such exposure just to be on the safe side.

Tricks to Pass a CBD Drug Test

In line with the issue of passing or failing a CBD drug test, it all comes down to finding ways of passing the test. First, passing the test depends on how well you research a CBD product before purchasing it. Don't be in a rush to buy a low-quality product with the hopes that you will save some cash. Go for a quality product that is pure regardless of the price.

Secondly, you should embrace the idea of asking questions about the CBD product. Find out the processing techniques that were used. This will give you a deeper insight into the product. You will be in a better position to understand whether cross-contamination might have occurred.

Third, always try to avoid being exposed to marijuana smokers for a prolonged period. This will help you eliminate any chances of failing a CBD test. Most importantly, get it clear that you cannot fail a CBD drug test if you are ingesting the right CBD that is THC-free.

Chapter 2: Methods of Usage and What to Use it For

There are several ways in which CBD can be consumed. Users have multiple options at their disposal to guarantee that they get the best results from the product. The common ways that will be discussed in this section include tinctures, inhalation, vaporizing, and topical applications. Each of these are effective methods of consuming CBD. Nevertheless, you should be aware of the pros and cons associated with each method.

Tincture Consumption

Tincture consumption is where the CBD product is delivered under the tongue. This is also referred to as sublingual consumption. Most tinctures that you will find in the market are vegetable glycerin or alcohol-based cannabis extracts. Often, they are of lesser concentration than the CBD oil. Tinctures are mostly available in dropper bottles. The concentrations of CBD oil within the products will vary. Some will be purely CBD oil, whereas others will have traces of THC. Be careful when buying them.

Since you will be carrying the product in the form of oils and tinctures, you might experience the disadvantage of fragile bottles. Therefore, if you are looking for a product that you can carry with you, oils and tinctures might not be preferable.

Ingestion

CBD can also be delivered to the body through the foods and beverages that you consume. Such CBDs are termed as edibles. These oils can also be added to coffee, baked goods, and smoothies. If you will be adding the oil at home, you should not overheat is, as this will cause an unpleasant smell.

Topical Applications

Topical products are usually applied to the skin. CBD topicals are known to treat arthritis, inflammation, sore muscles, and general pain. One striking aspect of topical CBD products is that they are non-psychoactive. Whether the CBD has traces of THC or not, they will not affect the brain in any way. As such, if you will be purchasing topical CBD products, you shouldn't worry about any psychoactive effects.

The advantage of using topical applications is that one gets to apply them to a particular area where the product should heal. However, the only likely disadvantage is that the application process can get messy.

Smoking/Inhaling

CBD oil can also be smoked. This is done with the help of an inhalation tool called a vape pen. This tool heats the CBD oil into vapor so that it can be inhaled. Inhaled CBD is quickly delivered to the lungs and therefore it has quick results. A major disadvantage of such smoking is that it leads to social stigma. People might end up mistaking your smoking habit if you will be using the product for a long period. Also, it is known to have negative health effects, particularly on the lungs. The other issue here relates to the size of vape pens you would be using. Often, these pens are not designed to control the amount of vapor you will inhale. Therefore, it could be a challenge for a new user to measure the desired quantity.

CBD Dosage: How Much Should You Take?

First-time users of CBD will have numerous questions about the product itself and its usage. Certainly, it is important to find out the recommended quantities of the product to ensure you get the best results. This is something that should be done by both experienced users and first-time users. With the uncertainty surrounding CBD oil, you can never be sure whether you are consuming it in the recommended amounts or not.

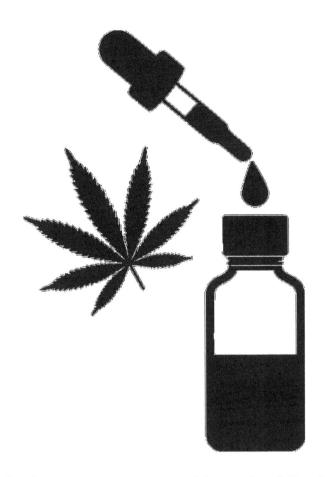

Obviously, there are numerous articles and publications that will talk about the health benefits of CBD. However, very few will take a look at its dosing. Combining this with the uncertainty surrounding the product, one could easily get confused. It should be noted that the FDA hasn't passed a recommended dosage that CBD users should stick to. Consequently, there is no official serving size.

The absence of dosage sizes from the FDA leaves people with the dilemma of having to guess the best dosage that fits them. Some rely on brands for information. Unfortunately, others are misguided by their friends who are completely unsure of how to use CBD for optimal results.

You might come across people telling each other that a dose a day is enough. Honestly, there is no clear way of defining the right dose that one should take. CBD users should, however, be keen on factors such as their weight, CBD concentration levels, their body chemistry, and the severity of their illnesses. In line with this, expect that you will go through a trial and error period to determine the best dose that works for you.

Choosing An Ideal CBD Dosage

The following are simple tips that should help you in settling for the right dose that suits you.

Use Your Body Weight to Decide

Your body weight will be a determinant factor in knowing the right dosage amounts to take. If you have a higher body mass, it means that you will consume more CBD. Having mentioned this, it would be best to consume 1-6MG of the product for every 10 pounds of your body weight. The following table should help you in finding the right dose that suits you depending on the level of pain you are experiencing.

			Weight:			
	<25 lbs	26-45 lbs	46-85 lbs	86-150 lbs	151-240 lbs	>241 lbs
Pain:						
None - Mild	4.5 mg	6 mg	9 mg	12 mg	18 mg	22.5 mg
Medium	6 mg	9 mg	12 mg	15 mg	22.5 mg	30 mg
Severe	9 mg	12 mg	15 mg	18 mg	27 mg	45 mg

Source: "What's the Best CBD Dosage? – CBD Origin – Medium."[19]

Know The Concentration of CBD Oil

The concentration of the CBD oil product will also have an impact on your level of consumption. Generally speaking, the higher the concentrations, the lower your intake. When buying any CBD from the stores, you should be careful to check the level of CBD concentration. Whilst doing this, you should ensure that you confirm the product is THC-free.

Desired Effects

Contingent on the expected effects, you will have to increase or lower the amount of CBD you deliver to your body. In this case, if you are suffering from chronic pain, you would consider consuming more. For mild pains, you only need to take small doses of the product.

---

[19] "What's the Best CBD Dosage? – CBD Origin – Medium." 24 Feb. 2018, https://medium.com/cbd-origin/whats-the-best-cbd-dosage-81ec4f95503b. Accessed 23 Apr. 2019.

Tolerance

With time, you might develop a tolerance to the CBD oil you will be using. When this happens, you may have to increase your dose to guarantee that you experience the anticipated results.

Talk to Your Physician

It is always advisable to speak to your physician whenever you are in doubt about a product that will have an impact on the health condition that you suffer from. Doctors with experience around CBD use will tip you on the best doses that will work for you.

How Much is Too Much?

There is always the question of whether one can take too much CBD oil. Considering the fact that CBD is non-toxic, you will not experience any negative effects unless you consume way too much. The good news is that research has shown that human beings are well tolerant of CBD. This means that your body would adjust accordingly depending on the levels of CBD you will be consuming[20]. You should also feel comfortable taking CBD, as there are no known statistics indicating that

---

[20] "2019 Ultimate Guide to CBD Oil: What is It? How Does ... - Joy Organics." https://joyorganics.com/ultimate-guide-to-cbd-oil/. Accessed 24 Apr. 2019.

CBD poisoned or led to the death of any individual.

Regardless, it should be noted that CBD should be taken by following the recommended dosages from your doctor. This helps a lot in preventing some mild side effects associated with the product. After knowing your right dose, you should stick to the dose unless your body gets to a point where it is tolerant.

CBD Side Effects

Certainly, it must have crossed your mind as to whether or not CBD oil has negative side effects. Indeed it is vital to find out whether the product has side effects before using it. It guarantees that you know how to deal with the possible side effects in case they ensue.

Bearing in mind that CBD is a natural product, there are a few possible side effects that a user could experience. Some of these effects include vomiting, diarrhea, dizziness, drowsiness, anxiety, mood changes, and dry mouth. The cannabinoid has lower side effects simply because it interacts differently with the brain receptors. Therefore, CBD lacks deadly side effects which are common in conventional medications.

Users should understand that the chances of getting addicted are low. The only thing that happens is that they grow a tolerance to the product and therefore, they might want to add more doses for effective results. When a user stops using the product, there are withdrawal symptoms that they could experience. Some of these include irritability, nausea, insomnia, hot flashes, and restlessness.

From the information on possible side effects, it is clear that there are no lethal effects of using the product. Regardless, this does not disqualify the need to consult a doctor before using the product. If there are other medications that you are using, it is vital that you find out whether the medications will react with the CBD oil.

Disorders and Diseases

Recent studies have shown the fact that medical cannabis has numerous health benefits to the body. In line with this, it is important to be aware of the common health conditions CBD oil is prescribed for. This information is important for those that would want to know whether CBD could be prescribed for them. The following is a closer look into some of these diseases and why CBD is a prescribed product for them.

Multiple Sclerosis

Multiple sclerosis is a disabling disease that affects the brain and spinal cord[21]. Symptoms of the disease vary considerably from one individual to another. Also, the severity of the

---

[21] "Multiple sclerosis - Mayo Clinic." 19 Apr. 2019, https://www.mayoclinic.org/diseases-conditions/multiple-sclerosis/symptoms-causes/syc-20350269. Accessed 23 Apr. 2019.

symptoms is distinct. Some of these symptoms include pain, vision problems, balance issues, muscle spasms, tremors, and numbness. CBD is known to help in reducing pain experienced when one is suffering from the disease.

Spinal Cord Injury

Trauma to the spine could easily lead to spinal cord injury. Such injuries could lead to complete loss of certain body functions. Spinal cord injuries are often associated with extreme pain. CBD oil can be used to treat such pain. Also, muscle spasms arising from spinal injuries could be treated by using CBD.

Arthritis

Basically, an individual suffers from arthritis when their joints are inflamed. Symptoms of arthritis are stiffness and pain in the joints. Unfortunately, the symptoms could easily worsen with age. Common forms of arthritis include rheumatoid arthritis and osteoarthritis[22]. The use of CBD oil is known to treat the pain experienced when one is suffering from arthritis.

Epilepsy

Epilepsy is a neurological disorder where the brain is largely affected. This leads to frequent seizures, unusual sensations,

---

[22] "Arthritis - Mayo Clinic." 7 Mar. 2018, https://www.mayoclinic.org/diseases-conditions/arthritis/symptoms-causes/syc-20350772. Accessed 23 Apr. 2019.

behaviors, and loss of awareness. Symptoms of epilepsy vary considerably. For some individuals, the symptoms could be mild whereas others could be severe. Seizures in different patients could last for a few seconds, whereas others could last for several minutes. CBD oil has proven to be an effective treatment for epilepsy[23]. This product helps a patient reduce the likelihood of experiencing seizures.

High Blood Pressure

High blood pressure is also identified as hypertension. High blood pressure occurs when the heart is forced to work beyond its normal rate. Hypertension causes the arteries to harden and could lead to serious health effects such as stroke, atherosclerosis, kidney disease, or heart failure. The use of CBD aids in lowering one's blood pressure. CBD could work as a vasodilator. It opens up the arteries, which prevents them from hardening. As such, blood flows without causing any increase in pressure. The best part is that CBD deals with some of the root causes of hypertension. It works by lowering the risks of obesity, reducing insomnia, and decreasing anxiety levels. These are some of the main causes that often lead to high blood pressure.

---

[23] "10 Most Common Conditions Medical Cannabis Is Prescribed For ...." 7 Mar. 2018, https://www.canabomedicalclinic.com/10-common-conditions-medical-cannabis-prescribed-for/. Accessed 23 Apr. 2019.

Diabetes

Diabetes is a disease which occurs when the blood glucose levels are extremely high. The sugar that you consume could lead to the disease. Insulin hormone works to ensure that glucose is consumed effectively by the body. When an individual suffers from diabetes, the insulin hormone does not function optimally. The absence of insulin means that sugar is not used by the body but rather it stays in the blood. There are two types of diabetes, Type 1 and Type 2. Too much sugar present in your blood can have adverse effects. Some of these effects include damage to your nerves, kidneys, and eyes. In extreme cases, it could lead to stroke and heart-related ailments.

CBD oil can aid in treating and controlling diabetes in several ways. First, it aids in preventing the occurrence of the disease. Equally, it helps in treating insulin resistance. This is because of its anti-inflammatory attributes. A reduction in inflammation of the cardiovascular and immune systems aids in ensuring that the body systems function optimally. Ultimately, this boosts the rate of sugar metabolism in the body[24].

Obesity is a risk factor that could lead to type 2 diabetes. Using CBD assists in preventing the risk of suffering from obesity. Therefore, in a way, it also helps in preventing diabetes.

---

[24] "CBD and Diabetes: 5 Ways Cannabidiol Can Help ... - Highland Pharms." 26 May. 2018, https://highlandpharms.com/cbd-and-diabetes-5-ways-cannabidiol-can-help-in-diabetes-management/. Accessed 23 Apr. 2019.

Chapter 3: How to Buy CBD Oil: Finding the Right Product

With the myriad of information about CBD over the internet, finding the right product isn't that easy. The CBD market has continued to thrive due to its associated health benefits. More and more people are out in search of natural remedies that have minimal side effects on the body. If you have never purchased CBD oil before, the information delivered in this section will help you make the right decision. This chapter will look at some of the most important details that you should look out for. Also, some of the top brands in the market will be mentioned to help you in making your purchase conveniently.

Packaging

When out shopping for your CBD product, the first thing that you will look at is the packaging. The packaging has all the information about the CBD oil you will be buying. You should be careful to notice anything that might not work with your body. You should check the packaging for CBD concentration. CBD oils are available in stores in varying concentrations. Don't just pick a bottle because it is labeled CBD. Confirm that the concentrations are suitable for your health demands.

Packaging will also inform you whether there are any traces of THC in the CBD product. Hence, this is a vital piece of information that you should not overlook. Before putting the product in your cart, you should have gone through all the necessary details to ensure you are buying the best product that serves you.

The other thing that you should look for when looking at the packaging is the ingredients list. This should be listed anywhere within or on the packaging. The absence of this vital information will certainly raise eyebrows.

Price of CBD

Another important consideration that should not be overlooked is that of price. In as much as you are looking for a quality product, it doesn't mean that you should be ripped off. Be careful to purchase CBD oil that is fairly priced. To ensure that you make the right decision, take your time to compare with other similar products. Ensure that you compare two or more CBD oils with the same concentration levels. If the price ranges within a particular value, it means that it is fairly priced.

Top CBD Brands

Besides focusing on price, you will want to mull over buying from the best brands in the market. Some of the best brands that you should consider going for include:

- BioCBD Plus
- Bluebirds Botanicals
- Charlotte's Web
- Elixinol
- Entourage Hemp
- Receptra Naturals
- Theramu
- Vape Bright

Buying from the best brands gives you some assurance that the product is of the best quality. However, this should not blind you from considering other essential factors.

Compare Strength

During your purchase, you will also want to compare the strengths of the CBD product you will buy. Check the labeling. Some oils will be labelled "full strength" whereas others might say "classic." A simple way of knowing whether they are strong or not is by dividing the milligrams (mg) concentration by milliliters of fluid or liquid.

Source of CBD Product

Another crucial consideration you ought to bear in mind is the source of the CBD product. Where is the oil manufactured from? Is it the USA or Europe? With the recent legalization of medicinal CBD, most brands have sprung up with all sorts of products. CBD oils that are highly recommended are those manufactured either in the U.S. or in Europe.

Flavor

Of course, the best CBD oil for you would be one that you can digest without feeling disgusted. Some manufacturers remain competitive in the market just because of the sweet flavors that they add to their CBD products. It is imperative that you choose a product that has a flavor that suits you.

Other Ingredients

Some CBD products that you purchase will claim to be pure. However, the truth is that most of CBD products are not that pure. They have other ingredients that you should consider looking at. In most cases, the common additives you will find are essential oils and vegetable oils. The best quality of ingredients would be easily noticeable. If you find trouble tracing the ingredients mentioned in the packaging, then you should definitely think of another CBD product. Don't settle for ingredients that you can't pronounce. If you notice anything that is not clear, simply look for another product that is transparent with its ingredient contents.

Health Claims

Another effective way of drawing a thick line between good and bad brands is by going through their purported health claims. Companies that place unreasonable health claims about their product are simply blowing their own trumpet. Claims purporting that the product works 100% should be considered as a red flag. Simply settle for a company that delivers without making any unproven claims about their product.

Quality Testing

The best manufacturers in the market would want to be sure that their CBD product is not contaminated. Also, they would want to know whether their CBD has any traces of THC. To achieve this, quality testing is imperative. Ideal manufacturers would, therefore, consider having their products tested to guarantee that they meet the quality standards required by consumers.

Go Through Reviews

An old trick that always works when shopping for things over the internet is going through reviews. Spend time reading through reviews that seem honest. The best CBD oil would be one that most people have left positive reviews about it.

CBD Oil Recipes

There are numerous stores that will offer you CBD oil at reasonable prices. However, one thing that you would want is something that you can digest with ease. This means that you would want to try out infusing it into chocolate bars, honey, caramels, lattes, and other treats. Without a doubt, this gives you a more personalized taste while getting the best from your CBD oil product. The good news is that there are several CBD oil recipes that you can try out at home. Some of these recipes are succinctly discussed in this section.

CBD Chamomile Tea Latte

Ingredients

- 2 Cups of unsweetened almond milk
- 2 tablespoons of maple syrup
- 2 tablespoons of loose leaf/ 2 chamomile tea bags
- CBD oil; 10 mg
- 1/8 teaspoon of ground ginger
- 1/8 teaspoon of freshly grounded nutmeg

- chamomile flowers

Directions

Start by mildly heating milk and tea in a medium-sized saucepan. Ensure that the contents do not boil. Remove the tea bags and stir in CBD isolate, maple syrup, nutmeg, and ginger. With the help of a blender, add some form to the content. This depends on your preferred amounts of foam. Lastly, garnish the top using chamomile flowers. Serve before it gets cold[25].

CBD Bliss Balls

Ingredients

- 1 cup macadamia nuts
- 1 tablespoon of melted coconut oil
- 1 teaspoon or 120 mg of CBD oil
- 1/3 cup almond flour
- ½ tablespoon ground cinnamon
- 1/3 cup of unsweetened shredded coconut
- 1 tablespoon of pure vanilla extract

---

[25] "CBD CHAMOMILE TEA LATTE - GOOD SAINT." 18 Apr. 2018, https://www.good-saint.com/recipes/cbd-chamomile-tea-latte. Accessed 24 Apr. 2019.

- 2 teaspoons of cacao nibs

Directions

Begin by placing the macadamia nuts in your blender for a few minutes. Leave the contents to mix until you obtain a thick paste. Add the CBD oil and the melted coconut oil to the mixture. Continue blending for a uniform mixture. Using a large bowl, combine the new mixture with unsweetened shredded coconut, almond flour, ground cinnamon, nut butter, and vanilla extract. Continue mixing the contents until you get a uniform mixture with a smooth texture. If you need the dough sweeter, add some drops of stevia. Throw in some cacao nibs and ensure they are evenly distributed. Next, scoop 1 tablespoon of the contents and roll it to form a small ball. Continue rolling until you finish the mixture in the bowl. With the mentioned ingredients, this should give you about 10 CBD bliss balls. Store your balls in a container and refrigerate for up to a week[26].

Evidently, from the recipes discussed, you are at liberty to bring in your creativity when creating your ideal CBD oil form. All of these should be done to make sure that you enjoy consuming the product. You should remember that there are many health benefits that it will have on your body. Therefore, consuming it regularly can help you ward off common diseases that have been discussed throughout.

---

[26] "Homemade CBD Bliss Balls to Help You De-Stress ... - Hello Glow." 23 Jul. 2018, https://helloglow.co/cbd-bliss-balls-recipe/. Accessed 24 Apr. 2019.

Final Thoughts

To this point, there is a lot that you have learned about CBD oil. The product has recently hit the headlines, but it doesn't mean that its use began yesterday. CBD use can be dated back to 6000 B.C. This was a time when human civilization was just beginning. With the advent of technology and prolonged research, people have realized that, indeed, CBD has numerous positive effects on the body.

Most people simply get confused about CBD oil. 'CBD' is an acronym that stands for cannabidiol. It is one of the compounds that is found in the cannabis plant. Mentioning cannabis gives one the impression that using CBD could make one feel high. This is not the case, from the information that has been discussed in this material. There is a thin line between the tetrahydrocannabinol (THC) and cannabidiol (CBD). Both are compounds found in the cannabis plant. However, they have different effects on the body.

CBD users ought to have it in mind that the product lacks psychoactive properties. On the other hand, THC does have such properties. It is for this reason that one should be extra careful when purchasing CBD oil from the stores. Some products could claim that they are THC-free when really they have a few traces of the component. Such CBD could pose particular negative effects that are linked to THC. Therefore, before pointing fingers at how CBD could make you feel stoned, it is vital that you be careful with what you purchase.

There are several diseases that can be treated with CBD. Some of these ailments relate to autoimmune diseases, neurological diseases, gut diseases, skin diseases, and neuropsychiatric diseases. Today, most people prefer to use CBD oil for pain relief. The main reason for this is that CBD oil lacks negative side effects associated with over the counter drugs. This makes the product fit for the body. CBD aids in pain relief, and it also helps prevent such pain from progressing. Its anti-inflammatory aspects help to free the body from pain.

If you have struggled with smoking for years, CBD is the product that you should purchase. CBD interacts with the endocannabinoid system and, therefore, it could help you quit smoking gradually. Of course, you shouldn't expect immediate results, but continued use of CBD in the right amounts will help you forget about smoking. Patients suffering from epilepsy should also turn to CBD for the best results. In fact, the government, through the FDA, has recently approved Epidiolex, a medicinal CBD which is used to treat complex symptoms of epilepsy.

Cancer is yet another major ailment that has robbed the lives of many people. Unfortunately, the existing methods of treating or preventing the adverse effects of cancer are costly.

With CBD, one can also prevent cancerous cells from migrating or growing. How is this possible? Scientifically, CBD aids in enabling antiproliferative, pro-apoptotic effects. These effects would work not only to shrink tumors but also to prevent the likelihood of cancer cells growing. Therefore, this should be taken as good news, as it could be a cost-effective treatment option for individuals struggling with cancer.

With the sedentary lifestyles that people have adopted these days, a regular CBD intake could help a lot in maintaining a healthy weight. Most people try over the counter drugs to reduce or maintain their weight, and they end up suffering from the side effects of such drugs. CBD oil lacks such negative side effects and therefore, it is a recommended product that will not only maintain your weight but also keep your heart healthy. It is a product worth trying owing to its numerous benefits that have been pointed out herein.

Undeniably, you have the freedom of choosing whether to use CBD oil or stick to standard pain medications. Nonetheless, it is worth noting that standard pain medications have serious health effects. Over the counter drugs such as aspirin, naproxen, ibuprofen and others could affect the normal functioning of your body. Prolonged use of aspirin, for example, could lead to the bleeding of your stomach.

More serious health effects could be experienced by those that take strong painkillers which are often referred to as opioids.

These are strong drugs, and thus they could cause cancer. Other side effects that one could experience include depression, dizziness, nausea, and addiction. So, as you aim to live a healthy and happier life, you should consider trying CBD over standard pain medications.

The legality aspect of CBD is another gray area that most people have not yet fully understood. CBD would be classified as illegal or legal depending on where it is extracted from. If the oil is extracted from marijuana, then it is not completely legal. If CBD oil is extracted from the hemp plant, then it is classified as legal. According to the government, the hemp plant has low THC quantities that would not be enough to intoxicate its users. Conversely, marijuana has high THC levels which are psychoactive. Accordingly, when purchasing CBD oil from the store, you should find out where it is extracted from. The last thing you need is to be in confrontation with the law without your knowledge.

The legality aspect of CBD extracted from hemp plant doesn't automatically mean that it will not appear on a drug test. It is vital that you understand the reasons why you could end up failing a CBD drug test. For instance, if you mistakenly buy a CBD product having THC, then you will fail the test. Also, the mislabelling of products in the market could have an impact on the products you will be taking home. Always ensure that you query about the presence of THC in the CBD product you might purchase.

With regards to usage, there are several options that are at your disposal. Some of the common ways of delivering CBD to your body include tincture consumption, ingestion, topical applications, and smoking. Each of these methods has its own pros and cons. It is essential to try out each and settle for the one that suits you. In terms of dosage, there is no recommended dose that is officially passed across by the government. Therefore, this leaves room for trial and error. Most users could end up relying on their uninformed friends to choose the right doses. This is not advisable. The best thing that you should do is to consult with a medical expert with experience on CBD use.

Essential factors to bear in mind when determining your doses include the fact that you should be aware of the CBD concentrations you are taking. If the CBD oil is highly concentrated, then you should lower your doses. Equally, your body weight could help you make the right decision. If you weigh more, you should consider adding to your dose. You will also have to reflect on the tolerance level of your body. If you use CBD for some time, your body could grow resistant. In such cases, you should add your dose for effective results. The exciting news about CBD is that it is non-toxic. Therefore, consuming too much might not necessarily have serious health effects on your body.

The side effects that you could experience by using CBD are simply mild effects such as mood changes, anxiety, drowsiness, dry mouth, etc. Don't expect to experience serious side effects like you'd get with other conventional medications. Also, there are minimal chances that you will become addicted to the product.

Important information that should be mentioned relates to the process of finding the right product in the market. With the vast number of brands available out there, a newbie could easily get confused about what is best for them. To circumvent this challenge, one should simply examine the packaging. Packaging will tell a lot about the CBD product. The labelling on the package will inform you whether the CBD is THC free or not. Also, it will inform you about its concentrations.

Going for the best brands in the market comes highly recommended. Most of these brands have passed their products through quality testing. Such testing guarantees that the product being sold is not contaminated. During your shopping, you should also be keen on the flavors that you pick. Choose something that you can digest with ease. In line with this, check whether there are any ingredients that might be harmful to your body. These additives are at times hidden from the user's eye. Avoid products that will hide the ingredient information from you. What are they hiding if they are sure of their product?

To sum it all up, CBD oil is a natural product that will help you live a healthier life by dealing with common medical conditions. Some of these diseases include diabetes, hypertension, obesity, insomnia, nausea, depression, and several others. Perhaps you might have tried over the counter drugs with no luck. Chances are that you could have suffered from its side effects and you are looking for a better option. CBD oil is the product that will help you forget about these diseases. It is legal and tested to the best quality to meet your health demands. Make the right choice today.

Bibliography

"10 Most Common Conditions Medical Cannabis Is Prescribed For." Canabo Medical Clinic. Last modified April 23, 2019. https://www.canabomedicalclinic.com/10-common-conditions-medical-cannabis-prescribed-for/.

"2019 Ultimate Guide to CBD Oil: What is It? How Does It Work? Joy Organics." Joy Organics. Last modified April 23, 2019. https://joyorganics.com/ultimate-guide-to-cbd-oil/.

"Arthritis - Symptoms and Causes." Mayo Clinic. Last modified March 7, 2018. https://www.mayoclinic.org/diseases-conditions/arthritis/symptoms-causes/syc-20350772.

Cadena, Aaron. "CBD Vs THC: The Difference Explained." Medium. Last modified September 30, 2018. https://medium.com/cbd-origin/cbd-vs-thc-the-difference-explained-b3cfc1da52f0.

Cadena, Aaron. "CBD101: The CBD Beginner's Guide." Medium. Last modified July 30, 2018. https://medium.com/cbd-origin/cbd101-the-cbd-beginners-guide-986274bbdf1b.

Cadena, Aaron. "What's the Best CBD Dosage?" Medium. Last modified February 25, 2018. https://medium.com/cbd-origin/whats-the-best-cbd-dosage-81ec4f95503b.

"CBD and Diabetes: 5 Ways Cannabidiol Can Help Diabetics." Welcome to Highland Pharms. Last modified May 26, 2018. https://highlandpharms.com/cbd-and-diabetes-5-ways-cannabidiol-can-help-in-diabetes-management/.

"CBD CHAMOMILE TEA LATTE." GOOD SAINT. Accessed April 24,

2019. https://www.good-saint.com/recipes/cbd-chamomile-tea-latte.

"CBD Oil: All the Rage, But Is It Safe & Effective?" WebMD. Last modified May 7, 2018. https://www.webmd.com/pain-management/news/20180507/cbd-oil-all-the-rage-but-is-it-safe-effective.

"CBD Oil: Uses, Health Benefits, and Risks." Medical News Today. Last modified July 27, 2018. https://www.medicalnewstoday.com/articles/317221.php.

Dadar, Areyo. "20 CBD Oil Benefits - Ultimate Guide on How to Improve Your Health." CBD Central. Last modified April 12, 2019. https://www.cbdcentral.com/cbd-ultimate-benefits-guide/.

"Hemp Oil Vs CBD Oil | What is the Difference?" Namaste.com. Accessed April 24, 2019. https://www.namaste.com/blogs/news/hemp-oil-vs-cbd-oil-what-is-the-difference.

"Homemade CBD Bliss Balls to Help You De-Stress Naturally." Hello Glow. Last modified September 8, 2018. https://helloglow.co/cbd-bliss-balls-recipe/.

"Multiple Sclerosis - Symptoms and Causes." Mayo Clinic. Last modified April 19, 2019. https://www.mayoclinic.org/diseases-conditions/multiple-sclerosis/symptoms-causes/syc-20350269.

PureRatiosHoldings. "The Brief History of CBD." PureRatiosHoldings. Accessed April 24, 2019. https://www.pureratioscbd.com/blogs/news/the-brief-history-of-cbd.

Made in the
USA
Monee, IL

15258216R00039